George E.  Waring

# The Sanitary Condition of City and Country Dwelling Houses

Second Edition

George E.  Waring

**The Sanitary Condition of City and Country Dwelling Houses**
*Second Edition*

ISBN/EAN: 9783337227159

Printed in Europe, USA, Canada, Australia, Japan

Cover: Foto ©Andreas Hilbeck / pixelio.de

More available books at **www.hansebooks.com**

# THE
# SANITARY CONDITION
OF
# CITY AND COUNTRY
# DWELLING HOUSES.

BY

## GEORGE E. WARING, JR.,

CONSULTING ENGINEER FOR SANITARY **AND** AGRICULTURAL WORK.

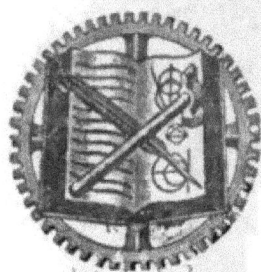

SECOND EDITION REVISED.

NEW YORK

D. VAN NOSTRAND COMPANY

23 MURRAY AND 27 WARREN STS.

1898

# PREFACE

## To the Second Edition.

---

The first edition of this booklet consisted mainly of a reproduction of two papers read before the American Public Health Association and the Public Health Association of New York, in 1876. These papers have been re-written, in the light of the advances made in the practice of House Drainage since that date, but their form has not been changed materially.

The paper on Country Houses led to a lengthy correspondence in the *American Architect and Building News*. This correspondence was reproduced, originally, as affording the best presentation of my own views on the subject, and as meeting objections which were likely to arise in the minds of those who had given it only casual attention. It remains unchanged in this edition; but it has acquired an added interest in the light of investigations which, since the date of the original publication, have led to the recognition of the agents which accomplish the destruction of organic matter, and to a more or less complete understanding of the conditions which may favor or hinder their operation. Although it is known now that the oxidation of the impurities of sewage in a surface soil is a bacterial and not a chemical process, the statements made as to the purifying capacity of the soil and the recommendations offered for the treatment of the hypothetical case under discussion need no revision.

G. E. W., JR.

NEWPORT, R. I., *October*, 1898.

# THE
# SANITARY CONDITION
## OF
# COUNTRY HOUSES.

THE sanitary defects of the average country-house are due to ignorance. Had the architect who built it been stimulated to learn what is required for a perfectly healthful condition, he would of course have been, in every case, vigilant to secure it. Did the physician know, except in a vague and theoretical sort of way—that is, did he fully realize—the degree to which the ailments he contends against, and which he should be vigilant to prevent, are diseases due to removable causes connected with the construction and arrangement of the dwelling, he would insist upon a reform.

Did the householder himself know the

extent to which his own efficiency and the health and lives of his family depend on an observance of the less obvious sanitary requirements, he would demand that both architect and physician should inform themselves as to the needs of his house, and should secure the fulfilling of those needs.

Fortunately, the crime of ignorance is declining. The technology of the plumber's art and the fundamental principles of sanitary engineering are more or less familiar to every newly fledged architect, and the physician has discovered that etiology and prophylaxis, too long subservient to therapeutics—are at least equal to it in importance. The householder himself, if he be of the more intelligent class, knows that obedience to hygienic laws is the price of safety, and he is willing usually to ask and to take advice from the priests and Levites of sanitation.

By far the greatest number of country-houses are farmhouses, laborers' dwellings, etc.; and these are not less subject to sanitary criticism than are those of the

better class, though their defects are
mainly of a different character, and relate
more to the grounds about the house and
to its water-supply, and to the condition
of its cellar, than to the arrangement of
its interior drainage. Indeed, in nearly
every case, these houses have no interior
drainage at all; and such reformation of
their character and condition as is needed,
will be sufficiently indicated in considering
the better houses. Unhappily, so far as
the occupants of the farmhouses and cot-
tages are concerned, there is little hope
that any considerable improvement will
soon be undertaken, or indeed that any
thing we may say here will be heeded.

It is sometimes hard to convince the
country physician of the older type that
his most important obligation to his community lies in a supervision of the conditions under which it lives ; but, until this
is done, it is hardly worth while to waste
breath upon the average members of that
community. We may accumulate evidence as to the fatal effect of prevalent
carelessness and filthiness in the cellar,

and in the soil about the house, until we are tired of making quotations; and, for every instance that we bring forward, of a death from typhoid fever traceable to the use of poisoned well-water, the farmer will produce a hundred cases of persons who have always used water from wells standing in barn-yards or close to privy-vaults or cess-pools, without suffering.

The action of poisoned water is less direct than that of a well-aimed rifle; and its effect, where there is any effect, is slower and less obviously connected with the cause than in a case of poisoning by arsenic. We can hardly hope to convince the common man of his error, and induce him to spend money, and to put himself to considerable personal inconvenience, to reform a state of affairs which has existed all his life-time, and which he believes to have answered well with him and with his fathers.

To his mind, typhoid fever, diphtheria, and the whole list of zymotic diseases, are afflictions sent by an inscrutable Providence for some hidden purpose of discipline; and he believes it his duty to bear meekly, if sorrowfully, the chastening to which he is subjected. He is still far from accepting the idea that his discipline may have for its direct purpose his regeneration in this very matter of hygiene. In their unvarying operation the laws of health (which are not entirely inscrutable) strike both the just and the unjust, and these laws are disciplinary, or not, according as we meet their requirements with intelligent obedience, or bow blindly and ignorantly before them. Typhoid fever does not come to us as a punishment for Sabbath-breaking, nor for profane swearing, but as a punishment for the one sin which brings us within reach of its scourge—the sin of unwholesome living. Then, too, sinners though we are, in this regard, it touches us so slightly—only here and there a case—that we are led, not precisely to run the risk of chances which we appreciate, but to remain placidly unconscious that the law is in operation about our own houses, awaiting only the due assembling of the conditions which bring its action to bear upon our own persons.

The great mission of enlightenment began its effective operations with the educated classes of society. Especially has it engaged the attention of the two professions to which I have referred. Within the range of these professions, the questions of healthful building and healthful living especially lie. From above, the enlightenment will be extended downward, until, in some millennial future, the merest cottager will understand the degree to which his health depends on the cleanliness or filthiness of his domicile.

In like manner, it is obvious that our efforts to secure an improvement in the construction and care of country-houses, must be first addressed to the more intelligent classes, and that they must work their way by example, among the poorer and the less informed. Let us consider therefore, by way of illustration, the case of an elaborate country-seat, built with a determination to secure every luxury and

every comfort, every convenience and
every safeguard, that the most skilfully
applied modern art can compass; a house
to which that compound adjective so dear
to the American heart may be applied in
every department from garret to cellar—
a house where everything is "first-class."

If we examine the old mansions of
our grandfathers, or go back still further,
to the seats of the nobility of past centuries in England, and compare our modern
houses with these, we shall realize what
enormous strides have been taken in the
improvement of many elements of our
building. Among other things, the modern mind has at last fully accepted the
fact that a wet cellar is dangerous, and is
to be, in all cases, and under all circumstances, avoided or abandoned. We are
still indulgent, and perhaps not very improperly so, of an occasional inroad of
storm-water, which subsides within a few
hours; but a cellar with standing water is,
at least very generally, *felt* to be an impossible accompaniment of healthful living.
By hook or by crook, we manage to get a

drain away from the lowest point of every
cellar dug in soil that *retains* water after
heavy rains We understand very well—
in the case of the better houses, perfectly
well—the importance of dry walls, at least
of dry interior walls. When we build in
brick or stone, our opposition to absorbed
moisture seems to stop at the point where
it is no longer injurious to wall-paper and
paint; but we do secure, almost universally, by the intervening air-space, a
separation of the wall next to which we
live, from the wall through which exterior
moisture penetrates. We have learned
how to warm our houses more uniformly;
and we realize, in far greater degree than
our fathers did, the importance of abundant sunlight.

But here, I fear, so far as health is
concerned, the improvement of our
building ceases; or, as we pursue our
investigations, we come to a point where
it seriously retrogrades. In the matter
of ventilation, our better-built houses
are often very defective. In our hot-air
furnaces we burn anthracite coal, separ-

ated from the air-chamber only by cast
iron, which is, especially when heated,
extremely porous to carbonic oxide. We
thus introduce an element of unhealthful-
ness throughout the whole house, which
constitutes, as compared with the influence
of the open fires of our ancestors, a very
serious defect. These influences, affecting
the wholesomeness of the air we breathe,
are serious; but they are far less so than
is our miserable system of house-drainage.

Half a century ago, in houses of the
better sort, the most active prejudice
existed against the use of any form of
indoor conveniences; and in spite of the
often dangerous exposure to the weather,
and of the universal stifling foulness of the
out-house, no one thought, except in case
of serious illness, of permitting defæcation
within doors. Partial invalids and delicate
persons must perforce subject themselves
to an injurious exposure. The objections
to this old system were extremely grave,
not only on the score of comfort, but
greatly also on the score of health. The
introduction of the water-closet marked a

real advance in our apparent civilization; and the general system of an interior water-supply and drainage, with the agreeable accessories of fixed wash-bowls, baths, laundry-trays, butler's sinks, etc.— of what the house agents call "all the modern conveniences"—have made life easier and more luxurious. In certain ways, too, they have added important sanitary benefits.

But in freeing ourselves from the prejudices of our fathers, and in gaining these marked benefits, we have exposed ourselves to dangers which are all the more grave because of their hidden and almost universally unsuspected character. It is by no means necessary that the introduction of modern plumbing-appliances into a house should be any thing but advantageous; but unfortunately, so little is popularly known of the sanitary requirements which should govern the work, while the influence of defective works upon the health of the household is of such a hidden character, that, in securing comfort and convenience, we have, in almost every instance, introduced a real element of danger.

We leave to the plumber, who, too often, is only a skilful mechanic, the entire control of the most important part of our house-building. It is true that, in the natural development of the art, and under the stimulus of severe criticism by engineers and sanitary inspection companies, the plumbers—of the better class—have improved their methods and their results greatly, and that many of them are entirely competent, and honest enough, to plan and execute well an elaborate system of plumbing. At the same time, this does not relieve from responsibility the architect who builds the house or the physician who has in charge the preservation of our health after we move into it. Both should qualify themselves, the one to secure and the other to maintain wholesome surroundings, by adding to their present work the most essential branches of sanitary engineering and sanitary inspection.

In a certain sense, the sanitary question reaches into a field where there is much uncertainty and speculation; but enough is already known concerning the relation between neglected or improperly controlled filth and the health of those who live subject to its influence, and enough is also known of the simple means by which all danger may be avoided, to make the prevention of diseases, arising from this source, practically certain.

Indeed, the effort to be put forth relates far less to the instruction of the architect and the doctor, in the very simple details of sanitary improvement, than it does to impressing upon them the importance of applying these details as one of the very first of their professional duties.

The precise methods of causation, and of propagation of cholera, diarrhœa, dysentery, typhoid fever, diphtheria, cerebrospinal meningitis, neuralgia, and the minor range of malarial fevers, it is the province of the physiological investigator to determine.

The understanding of these questions is not essential to the securing of healthful surroundings. It is sufficient for us to know the undoubted influence of neglected filth in either initiating or propagating all diseases of the class referred to, and the means by which the accumulation of such filth may be prevented. It is a matter of small consequence to the average house holder, who cares nothing for the general sanitary bearing of the question, whether typhoid fever is caused by the presence of some specific organism which is the germ of that disease and of that alone, or whether it is a modified form of a more common bacillus, which has gained virulence under certain peculiar conditions.

He does care very much, or at least he would care very much, if he thought any thing about it, that the condition of his house shall be in every respect such as to insure, beyond question the perfect safety of his family. He does not, it is true, realize the fact, which we fully appreciate. that his costly and finely finished water-works are a source of danger. He has trusted to his skilful architect to make sure that he is guarded against unhealthful influences from this source, as effectively as he is guarded against exposure to the weather. He has no time to devote to this part of his work; but he feels he has given it into hands fully competent to direct it, and he takes no further thought or trouble about it.

Unfortunately, so far as the question of health is concerned, he may have trusted the work to an artist, rather than to a sanitarian; for the architect, however competent to plan the general arrangement of the house, and to make it, without and within, beautiful, attractive, comfortable, and convenient, is—like the average owner— too often either ignorant of or indifferent to the requirements of the sanitary laws, as recently developed.

The owner takes possession of his new home, and subjects his family to unseen and unsuspected influences, which are quite likely, sooner or later, to manifest themselves in one form or other of ill-health. He then calls to his assistance a physician, who, perhaps, has applied himself far more to the art of healing, than to the art of prevention. In the slight ail-

ment, or in the grave sickness with which
he has to deal, he is skilful, useful, and efficient; but surely, physicians themselves
will confess that, as a class, they too seldom seek for the cause of ill-health in
conditions which are so universal among
their patients, and which obtain to such a
degree in their own homes, that they are
apt to be disregarded. He naturally looks
to some unusual condition, or to some unusual exposure.

Indeed, it is hard to realize that conditions under which the human machine so
generally works perfectly and easily, may,
under certain circumstances, become the
very conditions for the causation of diseases. If we can get doctors and builders
to *realize* the absolute, vital importance of
controlling the conditions under which we
live, we shall have done our best work.
Mr. Brown and Mr. Jones and Mr. Robin-
son—practical men, engrossed in the man-
agement of their affairs, and with a long-
cherished antipathy to theory and innova-
tion—will pay very little attention to what
we may say, or to any thing we may

write; but they will listen to the advice of their physicians, and in building, they will follow the least sanitary suggestion of their architects. Constant dropping will wear away even the stones of their indifference; and we shall, in time, secure a reformation of the whole community. But our earliest effect is surely to be produced by our influence over their professional advisers, who will, I trust, not misapprehend the spirit in which we venture to remind them of this vital and too little heeded element of their duties.

Let us come now to the specification of our charge against the quasi-modern country-house. It stands, we will suppose, upon nearly level land of a nearly impervious character; but ample provision has been made for the drainage of its cellar. Not far away from it, are cisterns and a well, each of which is in communication with the force-pump in the kitchen. This is provided with a twin cock by which water may be drawn from one or from the other at pleasure. Under the roof is a large tank, holding more than a day's supply; and this filled by the force-pump, furnishes all of the water needed for constant tap at every point. Near the middle of the house, one above the other on the different floors are placed the bath-rooms with water-closets and stationary basins—in the middle of the house, to be safe from the frost of more exposed positions. The attempted ventilation of these rooms is often only by a window into a closed well, or through a small register in the wall, opening into a small rough flue in the chimney, throttled from bottom to top with projecting bricks and lumps of mortar. The real ventilation is through the constantly open doorway into the interior passages of the house. In each bed-room, or in a closet attached to each bed-room, there is a stationary wash-basin, with its supply of hot and cold water. Under the staircase in the main hall, and often with no ventilation at all, are the conveniences of the master of the house himself. The butler's pantry has a sink connected with the main outlet-drain by a generous pipe. The kitchen sink has the same connection, and so have the laundry-trays, which, together with the servants' closet, are often near the level of the cellar-bottom—near the zero point of the drainage system.

The house has been built by contract; and a plumber, whose specification has related chiefly to the weight of pipe that he shall use, and to the character of finish of the basins and bowls, and their faucets and plugs, has been left to the exercise of his own discretion as to the arrangement of all the hidden parts of the work. His job is a satisfactory one, if the tubs and trays and sinks and basins have the proper neat look, and if an abundance of water is everywhere supplied, and everywhere flows readily away. For an outlet he has been provided with two cesspools; the first one, tightly cemented, has a trapped overflow; the second, receiving the overflow of the first, is built with uncemented walls; with a view to the percolation of its contents into the soil.

For a time everything works well; the clean new outlet-pipes perform their office satisfactorily, and the clean soil about the leaching cesspool absorbs the escaping liquid readily  The house is acceptable in every way; and its happy owner congratulates himself that he has secured all that modern art and knowledge can give him.

Let us examine this house after it has been a few years in occupation, with a view to studying its actual sanitary condition.  We will disregard, as foreign to our immediate subject, the flood of injurious carbonic oxide which its registers pour into its interior, and the said lack of ventilation which the substitution of the furnace, for the open fire, has inflicted. We will say nothing of the pressure of soil-water against the absorbent cellar-wall, nor of the damp emanations from the undrained, heavy ground around the house.  Let us confine ourselves only, and strictly, to the questions of water-supply and drainage.

The well, although perhaps not very near the leaching cesspool, and the now foul soil surrounding it, may get its water through some stratum of gravel which carries the ooze of this cesspool; or it may penetrate a permeable stratum, or a seam in the underlying rock, which brings it into communication with other cesspools or privy-vaults far or near. These impurities are not perhaps enough to produce an obvious effect, while the water in the well is high, and holds back the water in the soil as the land-water in the beach holds back the salt tide; but, when the supply fails, in time of drought, then the demand on the well is replaced by a flowing-in from the foul earth, and the impurities are concentrated to a dangerous degree. Or perhaps the dejections of a patient ill with typhoid fever, or other disorder of the bowels, have entered the stream oozing from the cesspool to the well. In either case, disease may follow. Warned by the frequent reports of diseases originating in this way, the master of the house has given strict and frequent orders that under no circumstances shall water from the well be used except for cooking; but some of the inmates, the servants especially, preferring the spark-

ling water of the well to that of the cis-
tern, bring the pump into communication
with the former; and now and then the
whole supply of the house, for a longer or
shorter time, is taken from this source.
Indeed, if there is a well in communication with the house-supply, it is simply
impossible to prevent the use of its water
from time to time.

The tight cesspool into which the drainage of the house discharges is of course
hermetically sealed, that there may be no
possibility of its emanations tainting the
air. It is connected with the outlet of the
soil-pipe by the best vitrified pipe, carefully laid. This pipe, for part of its
course, runs through soil that has been
excavated and refilled at the time of building; through soil, that is, which is sure to
settle as time goes on, bringing the weight
of the whole mass lying above the pipes
so to bear upon them as quite surely to
move them enough to open their joints,
allowing more or less of their contents to
soak away into the ground. Sooner or
later this leakage penetrates the founda-

tion walls, and taints the air of the cellar.

A strong, well-constructed four-inch soil-pipe descends from the trap of the highest water-closet, usually in a straight line, to the ceiling of the cellar, and passes in a straight course, and with a regular descent, to the point of outlet  It has been securely strapped to the floor-beams of the cellar, making it quite certain that a deflection in the main floor of the house, of even an eighth of an inch, will tear it loose from its attachment with the closet, and leave a little crevice for the escape of its gases, and of those formed in the cesspool.

The importance of ventilating the soil pipe having been recognized, a one and one-half inch lead pipe, leading from its highest point, has been carried out through the roof, closed over at the top to prevent the admission of obstructions, and perfor ated with a dozen little holes to give egress to the pent-up gases. This is not *ventilation*: it is only *renting*, only the re lieving of pressure, — an important office, but by no means a sufficient one.

The closets on every floor are of the "washout" type, shallow in seal; or—too often—of that ghastly foul sort which holds in a lower unventilated chamber nearly all that is admitted to them, save the water alone, until the solid matters, by decomposition, are enabled to pass away in a stream which was insufficient to flush them away as solids. The traps of the lower closets—too little air being supplied through the small venting-holes above the roof—are often emptied by siphon action, where a strong flow is rushing through the pipe from the emptying of a bath on a floor above.

To economize the work, or because no convenient course for a ventilating pipe can be found, wash-basins and other fixtures are set frequently on long "dead-ends" of nearly horizontal pipe, each a retort for the manufacture of foul and poisonous gases, which have no means of escape, save through the fixture, into the house, when the seal of the protecting trap is broken by siphonage, as is quite likely to occur.

In time, all the foul contents of the
cesspool, and the foul slime of the soil
and waste-pipes, having been for years
producing acrid gases, the leaden traps
under the closets, and the horizontal lead-
en connection-pipes have become more or
less honeycombed; and here and there
openings have appeared in the pipes.
These being in their upper sides, where
the usual plumber's inspection for leakage
does not detect them, they remain unsuspected, and they go on year after year
pouring out into the house their poisonous
exhalations.

The influence of even very small openings of this sort is far greater than would
be believed. I was told of a household in
New York which had long been a reliable
source of income to its attending physician. Upon his death, a younger doctor,
an enthusiastic sanitarian, succeeded him.
He soon became convinced that the illness
that had so long prevailed was due to em.
anations from the drainage-pipes of the
house. Plumbers were employed to make
a thorough inspection, and they reported

everything in perfect order. The cases
of disease kept occurring; and a sanitary
inspector from the Board of Health examined the house, and found no defect. The
character of the recurring ailments indicated so clearly a foul drainage cause, and
no other, that the physician finally applied
himself to a minute inspection of every
part of the work.

On the waste-pipe under a wash-basin
in a room communicating with the nursery,
he detected a very slight oozing of moisture, so slight that he did not feel sure that
it existed until he found that it moistened
tissue paper laid over the spot. The most
rigid scrutiny developed no other leak.
This pipe was taken out, and a new one
substituted; and, although he or his pre-
decessor had been called to attend some
member of this family almost weekly, for
a dozen years before, he was not called
again for eighteen months—and then only
because of the stork.

If any thing is certainly known with
reference to the house-drainage question,
it is that, in an unventilated system of

pipes, the foul matters which they contain enter into a putrefactive decomposition which produces poisonous, or at least injurious, gases; and, if any thing is clear to the common comprehension, it should be that pipes of a corrosible material—like lead—made by human hands and subject to the defects of all human work, containing, day and night, corrosive and injurious gases of this character, are dangerous inmates of any inhabited house.

Not only do these gases find their escape through defective joints, through perforations of old pipes which they themselves have destroyed, and through traps whose sealing-water has been sucked out by a flood rushing past them in the soil-pipe; but they have, as has been clearly shown by the experiments of Dr. Fergus of Glasgow, the power of passing almost unretarded and unchanged through the water seal-traps upon which we have so long depended with confidence.

Given the cesspool and the soil-pipe charged with injurious air, it is simply impossible that, under our ordinary methods of arrangement, this air can be prevented from mingling with that of our imperfectly ventilated sleeping-rooms and living-rooms. Every safeguard that modern experience has suggested should be applied from the beginning to the end of the system, to make sure that, whatever may be the character of the acriform contents of the pipes, they shall be strictly barred from escape into the house, and that every means shall be adopted to cause their escape into the free air above it.

Not only this, but every means should be taken to prevent the formation of these gases, and thus to gain the double security of their non-existence in their worst form, and against their entering our houses in their modified form.

And, first, for the prevention: Poisonous sewer-gas is a product of the obstructed decomposition of organic matter in the absence of light and of a sufficient supply of oxygen. In its most dangerous form it is believed to have but little odor.

If the decomposition takes place with exposure to a sufficient supply of common

air to furnish the oxygen needed for a
more complete decomposition, the gases
produced, although often more offensive
in their odor, are not only less dangerous
to health, but the more thorough decomposition is believed to be accompanied by
a destruction of the germs of disease.
These gases have in a much less degree,
if they have it at all, the power of decomposing lead pipes. In other words, this
worst enemy of those who live in modern
houses may be entirely or quite disarmed
by the simple means of supplying common
air to all parts of the drainage system.

To provide this immunity, so far as the
main artery of our works is concerned, it
is quite necessary to substitute for the pal-
try vent-pipe so often used, a pipe of
the full size of the soil-pipe itself, running
with the least and the fewest angles possible, quite up through the top of the
house. We must also admit at the lower
end of the pipe, a sufficient supply of air
—as copious as the danger of freezing in
winter will allow—to feed the suction, and
thus keep up a good circulation through-

out the whole length of the pipe. The effect of this ventilation should be made to extend as far as possible throughout the branches of the system; and with a view to this the water-traps, which, although they are not the most effective appliances in the world, are still sufficiently useful to be retained, should be placed as near as possible to the waste outlets which they are to protect. Where the outlet of a wash-basin, for example, is untrapped until the water-seal of a distant closet is reached, it becomes in time smeared for its whole length with the accumulated soap and filth of repeated ablutions; and these, although they are not what we recognize as fecal matters, are still organic matters of the same chemical character, and they produce in their decomposition, although in much less quantity, the same sort of gases.

Let every trap, then, be as near as possible to the beginning of each waste-pipe, and let the main soil-pipe be entirely untrapped, so that, as far as may be, every outlet drain in the house shall be in free communication with a thoroughly ventilated main channel. This secured, we may rest content in the belief that, so far as lies in our power, we have prevented the formation, anywhere within our drainage-system, of gaseous emanations which can be injurious to health.

The next step is to make sure that while we have, so far as is possible, disarmed our concealed but ever-present enemy, we bar every avenue to his nearer approach. He may perhaps no longer be dangerous: but we can never be quite sure of him, and he would be an offensive and disagreeable visitor. As a first step, in the place of strapping our soil-pipe to the beams of the cellar ceiling, let us set a stout post, bearing upon a firm foundation, directly under its bend, and so prevent the possibility of its settling a single hair's breadth. In this way we may keep a well-made joint with the water-closet trap perfectly tight. As a next step, we must either abandon all of our plumbing appliances, save only the necessary water-closets, and return to the old basin and pitcher, and the sponge bath or we must provide for the absolute and continuous sealing of every overflow and waste-pipe.

The ordinary water seal is a trap in more senses than one. Dr. Fergus found all gases with which he experimented to pass freely through its sealing water, ammonia passing through and reacting upon litmus paper in fifteen minutes. Furthermore, in cases where the trap is not frequently used, the evaporation of the sealing water leaves it open for the passage of air from the drain directly into the rooms. These defects are constantly present, even in the case of waste-pipes which are not subjected to pressure from the confining of their gases. Wherever there is such pressure, the evil is of course greatly aggravated.

The unquestioned advantages of a free supply of pure water in wash-bowls and bath-tubs on every floor of the house, can be safely secured only by some system which shall overcome their great defect, which far outweighs their advantages—the defect of affording a possible inlet to sewer-gas into the interior of the house. As at present constructed, it is safe to say that there is hardly a butler's sink, or a bath-tub, or a wash-bowl in use, which is not to a greater or less degree subject to this criticism.

The only *absolute* safety is to be sought in supplying a self-closing stop-cock to every waste-pipe or overflow-pipe, so arranged that it can be kept open only while it is actually held open by the hand. It is unnecessary to say, however, that such an arrangement would be extremely inconvenient. Traps are made which resist siphonic action, which contain a body of water too large to be lost in a short time by evaporation or capillary transmission through fibrous matters in the overflow, and which, at the same time, have their channels so arranged that the walls are well scoured at each discharge Even these are not wholly beyond suspicion. To those who have given no thought to this branch of the subject, it may seem a super-refinement of criticism to make this sweeping objection to an appliance of modern life which is in almost universal use in town and country; but I believe it to be susceptible of proof, that of all the causes of the various manifestations of impaired vitality which occur in our otherwise well-appointed houses, by far the greater majority have received their filth-born impulse from poisonous gases escaping through the overflow and waste pipes of wash-bowls, bath-tubs, etc.

Surely no one who has given attention to the details of plumbing can escape a certain sense of hazard, when he finds himself an occupant of a friend's guest-chamber, whose white marble fixed wash-basin whispers to him, the whole night through, of the hidden horrors of which it is the decorated outlet.

With a means for drawing water on each floor and with a closet-bowl through which to dispose of slops, the labor of attending our old friends, the bowl and pitcher, is not serious; and such an arrangement offers absolute security against a defect which has thus far not been remedied.

I have sufficiently indicted the very simply improvements that are needed in connection with the water-supply and drainage of that part of the house which is occupied by the family. The kitchen sink makes no slight demand upon our consideration. Its outlet offers a passage, not, it is true, for fecal matter, but for every sort of organic suostance from which fecal matter is derived; and which may supply, on its decomposition, precisely the gases which are generated in the ordinary soil-pipes. It does not carry the germs of disease; but its scraps of food, etc., are, on the other hand, mixed with congealed grease, which covers them to a certain degree against the access of oxygen, and tends to make their decomposition especially foul. Add to this the serious difficulty, that the congealing of the grease has a tendency to obstruct the waste-pipe, and lead to leakage and subterranean overflow of a serious character.

The methods for remedying these disadvantages are well known, and may be easily applied. The leading safeguard in the whole matter, here as elsewhere, is to be sought in the free ventilation of the waste-pipe at a point as near as possible to its source, and in the introduction of an efficient water-seal and grease-trap.

We come now to the method of finally disposing of the liquid waste of the house. Any one who has had much experience in the investigation of defective works must have reached the conclusion that those cases are really few in which even the defective methods adopted have been executed in anything but a defective way. The sanitary formula of Hippocrates, " Pure air, Pure water, and a Pure soil," is violated hardly less often by the earthenware drain without the house than by the waste-pipes within it. A vitrified earthenware drain laid on a firm foundation, and connected at its joints with good cement, is as perfect an apparatus for conveying foul liquids as we can well conceive of; but far too often the cementing of the joints is much less than perfect; and in almost a majority of cases, the pipe at some point rests upon new filling, which, by a settlement of a single half-inch, is quite sure to open a crevice at the joint, through which the trickling filth escaping from the house may find its outlet. In every case where it is necessary to pass through any thing but the original unbroken and solid earth, the excavation should be carried down to the undug bottom, and filled to the grade of the drain with well-compacted concrete. Either do this, or else substitute a stout iron pipe wherever new filling has to be crossed, however firmly this may have been packed.

The disposal of the liquid wastes of the house is one of the most serious elements of our subject. In a town, where we have a public sewer which may be depended upon for removing whatever we deliver to it, however defective this may be in the eyes of the public sanitarian, the problem is solved so far as the house-holder is concerned. He may easily make such a disconnection of the air-channel which brings his soil-pipe into communication with the public drain, as to insure himself against any danger from this source of poisoned air.

But in the case of a country-house, where a large amount of liquid is to be disposed of, and where there is a serious danger that we may contaminate the source of our drinking-water, or render the air about us impure, too much attention cannot be paid to the securing of a perfect method.

So far as I know, there are but two permissible devices in use. One of these, and the most objectionable, is an absolutely tight cesspool, well ventilated and accessible for inspection and cleaning, but from which not one drop of liquid can filter away into the soil—care being taken to empty it in such a way as to produce the least possible offence. Such a cesspool is a criminal—under restraint, it is true, but with a latent power for mischief which is appalling. Fortunately, it is no longer necessary that such a dangerous nuisance should exist, for even the smallest and cheapest house which has *any* adjoining plot of ground, even of a very modest size, can afford a satisfactory substitute.

The alternative is application to the soil. The upper layers of earth, to whatever depth air can penetrate freely, possess the power of destroying the dangerous and offensive properties of all dead organic matter which is brought into contact with them. Filth which is spread over the surface of the ground is changed rapidly into inoffensive mineral plant food and absorbed by growing vegetation. This change is brought about by biolysis, a form of oxidation similar in its results to combustion, but differing from it in this, that the agent which affects the chemical union of the oxygen with the integral elements of the filth is not fire, but myriads of microscopic living organisms, called bacteria. These organisms are to be found in abundance in every square inch of surface soil. Their function is to remove the wastes of life processes and to restore the materials of which they were composed to the storehouse from which

all plant life must draw. They are not
only beneficent; they are absolutely in-
despensable to the very existence or life
upon the earth; for without them the ani-
mal kingdom would soon be buried in its
own excretions, while the vegetable world
would suffer for lack of food. To avail
ourselves of their energies, we have only
to distribute the sewage over or in th·
surface soil, in such a way as to ensure
the intimate contact with the air of every
drop; and to change the point of application from time to time, so that the pores
of the ground may not become saturated
and thus closed to the entrance of air.

The simplest method of applying this
process is to flirt each pailful of sewage,
while fresh, over the grass, taking care
not to throw liquid on the same spot twice
in one day. In the elaboration of this
system, the sewage is collected in a flush-
tank, instead of a pail, which discharges
it automatically, at intervals, either over
the surface, or into open-jointed drain-tiles,
laid just below the surface. To secure

intermittent application, necessary for efficient aeration, the flow is delivered alternately to different tracts.

The area required is not large. One thousand square feet of lawn will purify the wastes of a small family. If a space of this size, at a little distance from the house, can be devoted to the purpose, the sewage can be run over the surface of the ground. Such a system is cheap to build, easy to control and efficient in operation. Where the only available land lies close to buildings, the sewage is discharged into open-jointed tiles laid a few inches below the surface. I know of one installation on the latter plan, in Newport, R. I., which has been in successful operation for many years, where the wastes of a large family are absorbed and purified by a small area of front lawn, lying directly between the house and the road. One end of the croquet-ground overlaps the disposal tract and hammocks are swung over the main distributing line of the irrigation tile. The flush-tank, built of white enameled

brick, which collects the flow and discharges it periodically, is in the side yard, not
far from the library windows.

This system of intermittent application
to land has been widely adopted for country residences and its use is extending
with great rapidity.

I am frequently asked whether the
earth-closet does not offer a solution of
the house-drainage question. Having
been for years its enthusiastic advocate,
and realizing as well as any one can its
value, under certain conditions, in the
hands of those who will give it a little intelligent care, I am still compelled to say
that, in the case of the ordinary householder, it is not to be considered where
the introduction of a good water-carriage
system is practicable. The latter requires
less attention, is more neat in some re-
spects, and can hardly become dangerous
even if neglected; but its chief value lies
in the fact that it will remove *all* the liquid
wastes of the house,—from the kitchen,
bath and wash-room, as well as from the
water-closet. These wastes require equal

care in treatment (save when the excreta
are infected with the germs of specific
diseases), for all contain the same putres-
cible materials. The earth-closet has a
field of usefulness,—to cover all those cases
where the water-closet cannot be used, or
where it would be subjected to the abuse
of ignorant or careless persons. Its value
for country schools and farmhouses which
are not supplied with water, and where
children or invalids must otherwise ex-
pose themselves to inclement weather,
cannot be overestimated. At the same
time, it is but a step in the right direction,
not a goal. It should be abandoned without hesitation wherever and whenever a
water-carriage system becomes possible.

My limited space will not allow me to
consider, as I should be glad to, the broad
and important question of the removal, by
underdraining, of the soil-water from retentive lands forming the lawns and gar-
dens of country-houses; and I believe
that the day has passed, when it is necessary to say a word on the subject of that
crowning abomination, the old-fashioned

vaulted privy. We still accept it as an evil which has too much headway for us to stop it at once; but those of us who have not been misled into the fallacy of believing that the "odorless excavating apparatus" has made its continuance permissible do not need to be reminded again of its entirely uncivilized character, and of the unhealthful influences that it must inevitably and in every case exert.

# THE
# SANITARY CONDITION
## OF
# CITY HOUSES.

A SUITABLY built, suitably arranged, and suitably surrounded city house is probably the safest of all human habitations; but a suitably built, suitably arranged, and suitably surrounded city house is probably the rarest of all human constructions.

The country house gets, from its isolated position, a full bath of sunlight, and a free circulation of pure air, which counterbalance many of its customary defects. But in spite of this, its defects are often pronounced; and deleterious influences arising from soil exhalations and from improper disposal of wastes are in its case often very serious.

A city house with an absolutely impervious sheet of concrete between its cellar and the underlying ground, with impervious cellar walls, with due protection against the rising of damp through its foundation, and with a sufficient circulation of fresh air through its cellar, is practically isolated from any source of danger connected with the ground over which it is built. The earth in front of it is covered with pavement, protected against undue saturation by its ability to shed rain; and the earth behind it is either covered in like manner with close pavement or has its exhalations filtered by the vegetation of its grass-plot — so that, supposing the whole area in its neighborhood to be protected in like manner by the belongings of other houses, there is little to fear from a malarious condition of the ground. Supposing every house in the neighborhood to be thoroughly well protected in the way indicated, it might stand over a pestilential swamp without much danger.

It is no argument against this assertion, that such of the houses with which we are familiar as stand over the site of an origi-

nal pond or swamp are subjected to malarial diseases, because the usual manner of
construction has left them without the
necessary protection against ground exhalations  Probably to a certain extent the
freest and best-drained soil acquires in
time, from the character of the early occupation of town-sites, a certain degree of
fouling which the absence of vegetation,
and the crowding of houses, so thickly as
to exclude sunlight and the circulation of
air, allow to become dangerous; and there
is frequently an undue amount of ground
moisture which affects foundation walls
and cellar bottoms as these are usually
constructed. The extent to which the unwholesome influence of the ground air
and moisture from the soil is felt by the
occupants of town houses varies, of course,
very much according to the original character of the ground. Where the ground
is dry and sweet there is little to be apprehended. The ordinary ventilation of the
cellar, which comes from careless workmanship, is generally sufficient for safety;
but in proportion as the dampness or foul-

ness increases, in just that proportion careless building becomes dangerous.

We know very well, from a difference in salubrity between houses standing on proper sites and houses standing on improper sites, that this influence of soil emanations is serious; probably, so far as the usual slighter malarial ailments are concerned, this soil influence is the most serious with which we have to contend. At the same time the debilitating effect of the exhalations referred to — headache, neuralgia, loss of appetite, intermittent fever, etc.—take a far lighter hold upon the popular imagination than do the often fatal diseases which are produced by bad air of another sort. The low condition and consequent susceptibility to infection which the malaria of damp soil produces, doubtless aggravate very seriously the dangers arising from the other source; that is to say, persons enfeebled by exposure to malaria would often succumb to infection, when a robust and vigorous person would withstand it.

Mankind has been too long accustomed

to living in the face of threatening infection, and has been too long educated in the belief that all fatal disorders are to be accepted as the chastening work of God's inscrutable purpose, for us to hope that the average man will at once realize the degree to which his life and health are dependent upon the manner in which he controls the circumstances and conditions of his living. Happily, it is now well recognized that typhoid fever, diphtheria, cerebro-spinal meningitis, and various grave disorders of the bowels, are the crop produced by planting in the system certain organic impurities, whose action is as direct, under favorable circumstances, as is that of the spores of *penicillium* in producing a crop of mould when planted on the surface of a damp boot. It is not necessary to discuss here the merits of the "germ" theory. It cannot be disputed that, whatever we may call the agent of propagation, there is an active agent peculiar to each disease. If we plant cowpox we grow cowpox, if we plant small-pox we grow small-pox, if we plant typhoid we grow typhoid; and so on throughout a long range of diseases whose limit is not yet defined.

Whatever our seed, our crop depends greatly upon the soil in which it is planted. In the case of a vigorous, active person, of strong constitution, and living under wholesome conditions, it may fall on sterile ground and be lost, while the same seed sown in the blood of the weakly may produce its fatal crop with certainty and abundance.

It is largely in connection with the influence of the constitution upon liability to infection—in addition to the minor disorders and discomforts resulting from the rising of swamp malaria and the conditions which produce fever and ague and neuralgia—that we have to consider the importance of excluding the ground air from the house. It is probably but rarely in city building that there remains in the subsoil such a degree of foulness as to produce typhoid fever and similar diseases; but the instances where a liability to fall before their attack is produced by this sort of unwholesomeness are by no means rare.

The causes of grave infection are precisely the same in the city that they are in the country, and they grow in both cases from improper protection against the emanations from the organic filth which is a necessary product of all human life. In the country it is perhaps less often by the fouling of the air than by the fouling of the water that these diseases are spread. In the city, the water coming from an untainted supply, the source of infection must be sought elsewhere.

We are far from possessing such accurate knowledge of the conditions of decomposition which favor the multiplication of the germs of disease, or the production of such a condition of the air as produces disease, that it can be demonstrated with scientific certainty that under such and such conditions typhoid fever will be produced, and under such other its production will be impossible. It is a case where we must consider circumstantial evidence.

No chemical analysis of the water-closet drainage, which oozed into the Broad

Street pump in London, demonstrates to us that germs of cholera were communicated to its reservoir; but it *is* known that a water-closet whose outflow reached that well was used by a cholera patient, and that within a week more than five hundred persons, scattered over one of the best parts of London, and even as far as Richmond Hill, whither they had fled to escape the plague, but whence they sent to this pump for water, were killed by cholera; the only possible communicating link between the individuals of this scattered multitude being that they drank this water.

We know by frequent observation, that persons living in houses where soil-pipes leak, or wash-basin traps are inefficient, are liable to fall sick with diphtheria or typhoid fever. We know that when the defective pipe has been removed and a tight one substituted for it, or when the faulty basin outlet has been closed, such diseases cease. We do not know precisely how the leakage from the imperfect pipe produced the disease. Therefore, all

that is said concerning this branch of the
sanitary subject, is to be taken as the sum
of empirical knowledge, and as being in
so far unscientific that our deductions are
not susceptible of clear demonstration.

Let us set aside the question as to the
manner in which zymotic diseases origi-
nate, and assume that it is demonstrated
that they are frequently caused by improper drainage, and favored by the admission of drain air into living rooms.
Taking this as a starting-point, we find two
most serious questions to be considered:

1. How shall we keep out of the house
the influences arising from the ground be-
neath it and beside it, which tend to produce a low condition of health, and to
create a susceptibility to zymotic poisoning?

2. How shall we protect ourselves
against such infection as comes to us from
within or without the house, as a result of
improper methods for the public and private disposal of the wastes of the body and
and of the household?

Concerning the injurious ground air, it

may be assumed, however serious the difficulty, that it may be nearly or entirely remedied by a thorough draining of the soil below the level of the house cellar, by making the cellar-floor, the foundation-walls, and the pavement and walls of basement areas, hermetically tight; and by providing for the complete, even if very slight, ventilation, of the cellar itself. This is recognized on all hands, at least so far as the cellar wall and foundation are concerned, as being necessary to the best building. In time it will come to be absolutely required by public authorities who have the regulation of the way in which builder's work must be carried out.

That the importance of this complete separation of the house from the ground under and about it is by no means popularly regarded as essential, our daily observation proves. Those contractor-built rows of cheap houses, built by the block and sawed off in sixteen-foot lengths to suit the demand, which cover so many hundred acres of every great city, are built almost invariably without the least regard to the influence of the soil below them upon the health of those who are to live within them. That strictly American adjective, "first-class," which makes every degree of badness acceptable to the ambitious mind, has its requirements fully satisfied by a certain conventional expenditure about the front and the entrance door of the building, by high ceilings, and by a judicious touch of "Queen Anne" joinery and paper-hanging. The house may be the veriest rattle-trap that ever trembled over the site of a recent swineyard; there may be the freest racing-ground for rats from garret to cellar; it may have twenty openings in its drainage system, which are separated from the street sewer only by ineffective and often inoperative water-seal traps; its foundation walls may leak, and its cellar may often hold stagnant water. With all these defects, and with all the "scamping" of its work, which are evident to the practised eye, if its experienced builder has had the shrewdness to give it that touch of cheap finish which makes it "first-class," he may count on a price that will make his operation a good one. Should he be able to add the taking recommendation that the house has been built "entirely by days' work," it matters little that it was the days' work of apprentices and bunglers.

One of the almost universal defects of New York houses is strictly fundamental. The proportion of houses of the costlier sort that would bear a rigid inspection as to the efficiency of their cellar floors, foundation-walls, and areas, must be extremely small. The gravity of this drawback is sufficiently understood by all who know the prevalent ailing condition of the women and children whom these houses shelter.

Much more serious, when measured by the death and pain that it produces, though hardly more so with regard to its effect on the health and efficiency of the people, is the question of disposing of the household wastes.

Men living in widely scattered communities find it easy, in their rude way, to get rid of the organic refuse that they produce, without serious injury to their health. As houses are made tighter and more gathered together, the trouble increases with regard both to the waste of each household as reacting upon its own members, and to the influence that it may have upon the members of other households. When men gather together into closer built towns, they bring with them at first the institutions of the village —the vault in the back yard, the leaching cesspool, and the slop-gutter. The methods of life implied by the use of these systems are accompanied by defects of construction and ventilation which give a high death-rate. It may be questioned whether, with a public supply of good water, there is any great amount of actual poisoning occasioned by such disposal of filth. Indeed, the statistics of health in Baltimore show an exceptionally small death-rate, although the slop-water of the house is carried away through surface channels, and the gutters at the sides of the streets are almost constantly running with soap-suds and kitchen sink waste. The untidiness suggested by this custom makes it one of the first efforts of the dainty and fastidious to hide such matters out of sight, by passing them away in covered channels.

Human ingenuity has been able as yet to devise no system for the disposal of all manner of liquid waste which is at once so inoffensive, so invisible, and so healthful, as a well-arranged system of water-carriage removal. The unfortunate thing about it all is that it is easy to meet the requirements of the fastidious by such a development of the system as is, from a sanitary point of view, the worst possible. Marble-top wash-stands with silver-plated fittings, decorated china closet-bowls, porcelain-lined baths, stationary trays in the laundry, and the brightest and handsomest workmanship wherever the plumbing is visible throughout the house, are too often the outward manifestation of pestilential hidden dangers.

Art can hardly achieve more in the way of luxurious appointments than is compassed by all of these details in a modern house of the best sort. The character of

their finish has much to do with the estimate that the intending purchaser or tenant puts upon the house he examines, as
they are the subject of some of the most
minute of the architect's specifications.
When we consider the interior construction and arrangement of the hidden system to which they belong, we approach a
part of the subject concerning which the
purchaser, the architect, and the tenant,
are too often ignorant and indifferent.
Nor do the dangers which belong to the
modern house drainage system cease when
we pass the limit of private work, and
come to the public sewer to—and from—
which the house drains lead.

The sewer and the drain meet one im-
perative requirement of the community.
They are hidden from sight, and their
processes are not offensively manifest, as
are those of the slush-bearing surface
gutter.

It is often assumed, perhaps because of
the name given to the air of which we
hear so much and which is so widely destructive—" sewer-gas ", that the diffi-

culty lies entirely or chiefly in the public
sewer, and that we have only to improve
the character of this, or so to detach our
private system of drainage from it as to
prevent the transmission of its air.

City sewers are too often badly planned,
badly built, and badly kept, and they do
unquestionably produce a vast amount of
disease and death. We can by no means,
however, charge them alone with all or
nearly all of the harm that is done; for so
far as the production of dangerous gas is
concerned, the waste-pipe of the house itself, smeared from top to bottom with the
foulest organic matter, putrefying often
under the worst conditions, and with frequent variations of temperature caused by
the entrance of hot and cold water, is at
least a brave rival of the worst street
sewer.

There are still many houses in all our
cities in which lead soil-pipes are used.
The experiments of Dr. Fergus, of Glasgow, have demonstrated in the clearest
way the great suspectibility of lead to the
corroding influences of foul gases arising

from organic decomposition. He cites a great number of instances in which even after a few months' use the action of these gases upon the material of the soil-pipe has perforated it through and through, and in some cases completely honeycombed a considerable area of its wall. This effect is produced by gases and not by the foul water, as is proven by the fact that the perforations are always at the upper side of the pipe, and never on its lower side, where the water flows. It occurs along the upper side of horizontal and oblique pipes, and especially at the upper side of a bend, as in front of a trap; for the reason that the lightness of the gas causes it to lie chiefly against these parts of the pipe. The perforations being at the upper side of the pipe, they are not manifested by the leaking out of water, as the conduit is rarely filled. Often where it is horizontal or oblique, it serves only as a gutter, its upper side being largely eaten away.

Even the smallest perforation may become a source of the most serious danger;

a mere pin-hole may permit the escape of such an amount of air from the pipe as to poison the atmosphere of a large room. The apertures formed by corrosion, however, are rarely so small as pin-holes, and they are not infrequently large enough to admit the finger.

In modern practice it is practically universal to use for the soil pipe and the larger branch-wastes, cast iron in the place of lead. This material is not susceptible to perforation from the action of its contained gases, but, as drainage works are constructed, it is often fed by numerous waste-pipes of lead; which come to it from bath-tubs, wash-basins, butler's sinks, laundry trays, and urinals, and even the water-closet often has a trap or a connection pipe of lead. All of these leaden connections are subject to the same liability to corrosion as is the lead soil-pipe itself; and in one sense they aggravate the danger, from the fact that perforations occurring in them are more likely to discharge gas into sleeping-rooms or into the more frequented parts of the house.

The especial adaptation of lead to the construction of these minor waste-water channels because of its flexibility, and of the ease with which it is jointed, make it almost necessary that it should be used; but, as plumbing-work is generally constructed, it is used with more or less risk.

Abundant ventilation of the entire drainage system is most important.

The poisonous sort of sewer-gas is the product of an obstructed decomposition; of fermentation, which Pasteur aptly calls "life without air." The atmosphere within the unventilated soil-pipe does not contain sufficient oxygen to supply the continuous decomposition, which is thus checked until the oxygen which it requires is supplied by constituents of the organic matters themselves—a process which leads to a radical difference in the resultant gases. Instead of being a thorough destructive oxidation of the material it becomes a putrefying decomposition, producing foul smelling and dangerous results.

That part of the soil-pipe which carries the waste of the butler's pantry and the kitchen sink, is more or less charged with melted grease, which coats the accompanying particles of food and of filth, and so shelters them from the action of the air, giving the same pernicious character to their decomposition.

The most important improvement in house-drainage ever made is one which grew out of our better knowledge of the true character of the decomposition taking place in the soil-pipe. It has for its objects—and it accomplishes these objects perfectly—the reduction of putrefactive fermentation to the minimum, and the complete and immediate dilution of the gases which the slight remaining putrefaction does produce. It consists in creating throughout the whole length of the soil-pipe a constant supply and a constant movement of fresh outer air. This is accomplished by providing a fresh air inlet at the lower end of the soil-pipe, at or near its passage through the house-wall, and the continuing of the soil-pipe itself, full bore, up through the roof of the house to a point well above all windows.

The soil-pipe being properly constructed and duly ventilated, the only further practical improvement in the waste drain system seems to lie in making its branches, which lead from bath-tubs, wash-basins, etc., as short as practicable. Unless very short, each of these lines should be ventilated independently.

The layman in sanitary matters usually considers that the larger the diameter of the waste-pipe the less the danger of obstruction. The fact is that all increase above a certain size—smaller than the size in average use—is a distinct detriment. This is especially true of the waste-pipes from kitchen and pantry sinks. Experience has proved that large pipes choke frequently because the stream flowing through them has not sufficient force to keep them clean. With a flow of low speed, grease, which a strong flush would carry to the outlet, is deposited upon the walls, layer upon layer, until the water way is restricted to a size which gives the current a scouring velocity. The channel is then no larger than that of a small pipe, but it is tortuous and foul. At any moment a portion of the grease, breaking up under the action of putrefactive agencies, may become detached and cause complete obstruction. A pipe of such size as to maintain from the first a cleansing velocity would remain smooth, true and unfouled. A diameter of one and a quarter inches is amply large for the waste from a kitchen sink. Indeed, I should not hesitate to use a one-inch pipe for this purpose.

The essentials of a good water-closet may be enumerated, in the order of their importance, as follows:

There must be no valves, plungers or moving parts in the bowl or in the course of the outlet. It is hardly necessary to say that the "pan closet"—the Devil's vinaigrette—which was once in almost universal use, is absolutely inadmissible in modern plumbing. It is offensive and unsafe. The few that remain in service cannot be banished too quickly. All other closets which have moving parts share, to a greater or less degree, the same objections

There must be a reliable seal, deep enough to withstand considerable pressure and not susceptible to siphonic action. It is better that this seal should be in the bowl, in plain sight, rather than concealed under the floor or in the body of the closet. The depth of seal and the cleanness of the sealing water will then be apparent to every one.

There must be an abundant supply of water at each flush; not merely enough to drive excreta and paper promptly out of the closet, but sufficient to lubricate the walls in advance and to scour them after the passage of the foul matters, and copious enough to carry its burden to the ever-moving stream in the street-sewer. The flush should be from a box-tank,—not directly from the pipes of the main supply. It should discharge a fixed quantity quickly, regardless of the length of time that the chain is held, and it should have an "after-fill" device which will fill the trap of the closet to the overflow point.

The bowl should hold water sufficient

for the complete submersion of deposits. This will minimize the odor resulting from its use.

The closet should be set without casing or concealment of any sort, on a durable impervious floor, preferably white, with white surroundings, so that every particle of dirt may be painfully apparent. The seat should be as small and light as possible,—a single piece of wood with a hole in it, resting directly on the bowl and hinged so that it may be turned back. No cover is needed or wanted. The entire apparatus inside and out, should be open to air, light, cleaning and the unbidden inspection of all who come within sight of it.

Stationary wash-stands—and all other fixtures connected with the drainage system of a house—should be kept out of and away from sleeping-rooms. Their proper place is in bath-rooms and lavatories. These should have abundant outside ventilation and spring doors separating them from the rest of the house.

Neither basins, baths, sinks or laundry tubs should be encased, but each should stand open to ventilation and to view. The waste from each fixture must be trapped, as close to the fixture as possible, by some approved deep-seal trap, secure against siphonic action.

Fixtures with concealed overflows are to be avoided, for these hidden passages become fouled with soapy matters and it is difficult to cleanse them. A satisfactory device which overcomes this objection, and which at the same time obviates the use of the nasty chain and plug, formerly so common, is the "standpipe overflow." This is simply a short pipe, with one end ground to fit the outlet, which serves both as plug and overflow. It can be cleaned most readily.

There are many minor details that might with advantage be alluded to did time permit—such as the objections to long horizontal waste-pipes; the importance of having these waste-pipes trapped only at their upper ends, delivering at their outlets into a freely ventilated soil-pipe; the increasing importance of ventilating the waste-pipes in proportion as their length increases; the necessity for delivering the ventilation of foul pipes at such points as will prevent their outflow of air from being involved in the back-draught of unused chimneys; and all the long detail of house ventilation; also the pregnant subject of the poisoning of the air by the carbonic oxide produced by the burning of anthracite, which Dr. Derby demonstrates in his valuable monograph on "Anthracite and Health;" together with the effect on health of that foul smelling effluvium which comes from the heating of organic dust by steam-pipes, and which makes an unventilated, steam-heated room so disgusting to the unaccustomed nostril.

These are relegated to a secondary position because, like the necessity for free sunshine in all inhabited rooms, they are less obviously connected with the question of life and death than is the matter of drainage pure and simple, and are therefore less likely to engage immediate attention.

Interest in sanitary improvement will

naturally first apply itself to the more serious causes of fatal and distressing disease; but once awakened it will pursue the whole range of the subject, and will, let us hope, not abate until it has compassed a perfectly wholesome condition in every department, and has secured to all, what all have a right to demand, an entirely safe human habitation.

# EXTRACTS FROM CORRESPONDENCE

IN THE

American Architect and Building News,

ON THE

# DISPOSAL OF THE LIQUID WASTE

OF

COUNTRY HOUSES.

# CORRESPONDENCE.*

*December* 16, 1876.

I HAVE followed with much interest the series of articles you have published on " The Sanitary Condition of Country Houses," the subject being one to which I have given considerable attention.

It approaches, but does not quite reach, one of the points involved, which is of so much importance, that I venture to ask for the consideration in a subsequent paper. The question I refer to is that of the disposition of sewage from a country house, where there is no town drainage available, and *where the grounds surrounding the house are level* (which, by the way, is the usual condition in country towns). To simplify the consideration, let it be supposed that there is a street water-supply,

---

* "T" is HENRY R. TOWNE, Esq., of Stamford, Conn. "B." is JAMES BAYLES, Esq., of New York City. "W." is the writer of the foregoing pages.

so that contamination of springs is not to be guarded against; that the house is provided with water-closets, sinks, etc.; that the waste-pipes are all connected with four-inch iron soil-pipe, and that the latter passes through the basement wall, from three to four feet below ground, to avoid frost. Now, given the above conditions, how far must the sewage be carried from the house, and how shall it then be disposed of?

Obviously the character of the soil is an important element; and I would suppose, therefore, the two most ordinary cases, (1) where the soil is of gravel, porous; and (2) where it consists of clay, not porous. It should be remembered, also, that the soil-pipe necessarily leaves the house at a depth which precludes the subsoil irrigation system of Mr. Moule.

The conditions I have supposed are such as will apply to the majority of residences in small towns and suburban villages, as well as to many country houses; and you can do no more useful service than by indicating the proper treatment of this problem, which, perhaps on account of its difficulty, is oné but very slightly touched upon in most treatises on sanitary engineering.

T.

---

December 23, 1876.

IN the communication published in your issue of Dec. 16, a question is raised as to the disposal of the liquid wastes of houses which stand on level ground—the usual condition in country towns. Mr. Towne thinks that the directions contained in my address before the American Public Health Association do not quite reach this point.

I see no escape, in the case of such houses, from the necessity for making the conditions conform to the requirements. Certainly the requirements cannot be made to conform to the conditions. The production of liquid wastes which are sure to endanger health if not properly got rid of, is a necessary part of the economy of every household. So far as I know, there

are only five systems by which this liquid
can be treated.

1. By discharge through an open surface gutter to a distant open vat, or waste
corner of the grounds. This is the most
offensive system, and the one least likely
to be adopted by persons who are at all
nice in their ideas of decency; but it is
not necessarily dangerous to health, if the
final deposit is at some distance from the
house. If the gutter is kept well slushed
out, the decomposition at the distance ter-
minus will have its foul emanations so diluted by the air before they can reach the
windows as to be innoxious—save for their
smell. Happily the sense of decency will
prevent the adoption of this tolerably safe
but entirely nasty expedient.

2. By discharge into a leaking cesspool. This is the most dangerous system
yet devised, especially for houses not supplied with water from public works. It is
also a system which public opinion and
public authority must soon prohibit. The
covert poisoning of the ground from which
the water-supply of a whole neighborhood

is taken, and from which the "ground air" rises into and around human habitations, will not much longer be permitted. So far as the house itself is concerned, there exists the further defect of a constant formation of sewer-gas in the cesspool, which has no outlet save back through the pipe leading from (and to) the house —a channel of communication which no form of water-seal trap can close.

3. A tight cesspool; not simply a "cemented" cesspool, but one which is known to be, and is sure to remain, absolutely tight. It is possible to make such a cesspool as this, but it is not usual; and it is possible, but it is still more unusual, to ventilate it so that the formation of poisonous gases need not be feared. In its most perfect condition it is subject to the necessity for frequent emptying; and is sure to be at best only a mitigated nuisance, ready to become a source of real danger whenever its impervious wall is accidentally made pervious, or when its ventilation fails from any cause, or when its proper emptying is neglected, or when

a sudden storm causes it to overflow, or to set back into the house-drain. Under the best circumstances and conditions, such a cesspool may be permitted; but when the householder himself is not constantly vigilant and attentive—even anxiously so—it may become a cause of serious mischief.

4. By discharging into a public sewer. If this is well contrived, well constructed, *and well ventilated*, it offers the best solution of the problem, so far as the individual householder is concerned.

5. By discharging the liquid waste of the whole house (through suitable flush-tanks and settling cisterns) into a system of sub-irrigation-pipes as described in the paper which suggested Mr. Towne's letter. Where the public sewer is not available, I regard this as much the best device of all.

I see no escape from such conditions as the above paragraphs indicate as necessary under one system or the other. With a public sewer, the soil-pipe may of course leave the house at a depth of four feet or more. If the tight cesspool is to be used, it may be placed so far underground that the same depth will be admissible; but my advice would usually be against providing for any such accumulation of putrefying filth. The sort of gasometer that the dome of such a cesspool would furnish ought not to be an adjunct to any habitation.

If the sub-irrigation system is to be used, then the grade must be made to conform to it: that is all there is about it. The soil-pipe cannot leave the house at a depth of four feet below the level of the ground to be used.

Fortunately this is not necessary. The *ground* may freeze to a depth of four feet; but a soil-pipe drain carrying the warm outflow of the house would not freeze at a depth of two feet, probably not at considerably less than that. My own house-drain is only two feet deep. and has remained unaffected when the ground was frozen solid nearly five feet deep. My irrigation-drains have worked perfectly in the coldest weather, at a depth of one foot. My flush-tank stands mainly above ground, outside of the house, and is only protected by a one-inch board "dog-house" packed with leaves.

These facts indicate that much less depth is needed than Mr. Towne suggests. And the fact is that very few places, even in villages, are *level:* there is usually a slight fall, and a slight fall is all that is needed. Whatever is needed *must* be furnished either by raising the house, by lowering the ground, or by adjusting the level of the pipes to suit the conditions. Ordinarily a little skill and ingenuity in such matters will suffice to accomplish this. I have not as yet met a case where there was any serious obstacle to be overcome.

W.

---

*January* 13, 1877.

MR. WARING'S reply to my query, as to the best mode of disposing of the sewage of country houses which stand on level ground, is interesting, but by no means exhausts the subject.

Of the five systems Mr. Waring enumerates, the first, second and third, are practically excluded from consideration by him on account of their objections, and the fourth (the use of a public sewer) is excluded by the conditions supposed in my query, so that only the fifth (the sub-soil irrigation system of Moule) remains; and to this Mr. Waring nails his colors with the remark that if the grade does not admit of this system it "must be made to conform it: that is all there is about it."

This position I think is hardly tenable, however, for in many places the grade is uncompromisingly and provokingly level, and *cannot* be altered, as, for instance, in such districts as Central New Jersey, where in some towns and villages the grade does not vary twenty inches in the whole place, let alone within the bounds of an ordinary house-lot of say fifty by one hundred and fifty feet. In such cases the sewage *could*, of course, be collected in a tight cesspool, thence pumped into a raised flush-tank, and then discharged in sub-soil irrigation pipes: but this plan is too expensive, both in first cost and in operation, to admit of general application, and is moreover open to the objections Mr. Waring makes to tight cesspools. And thus, *for flat grounds*, system number five is also in many cases excluded.

If the question of cost be ignored, there is little difficulty to the engineer in dealing with the problem we are considering, under any conceivable circumstances; but it must be remembered that cost is almost invariably an important if not a controlling element, and the question therefore is: How, at reasonable cost, can we secure the best results?

Now I believe that where, as I have supposed, there is a street water-supply so that we need not fear contamination of drinking-water, the leaching cesspool *properly used* may, notwithstanding its conceded objections, be our best reliance. The condition under which it may be resorted to, I conceive to be as follows: It should be located as far from the house as possible, but not less than fifty or sixty feet, and should be carried to a depth of at least four or five feet below the mouth

of the discharging sewer. Its diameter
(as dug) for an ordinary dwelling-house
should be at least ten feet; and its walls
of large, loosely fitted stones, should be
" drawn in " from a point just above the
sewer outlet as quickly as practicable, so
as to form a dome entirely covering the
cesspool, above which, to the ground
level, the excavation should be filled in
with clean earth in which vegetation
should be encouraged.

Before closing the cesspool, two four or
or six inch pipes of lead or galvanized
sheet iron should be laid in place, one
reaching down almost to the level of the
sewer, and the other starting from the apex
of the dome. These pipes should be led
below ground to some convenient point,
and then carried to an elevation of at least
eight or ten feet above ground, and then
capped with ventilating cowls, the one
leading from the top of the cesspool having a cowl so constructed as to create an
upward current in the pipe, the other having a reversed cowl, like a " wind-sail,"
which will force air downward into the

cesspool. By this means we prevent any pressure within the cesspool or sewer from the formation of gases of decomposition, and also provide for a circulation of air within the cesspool which will constantly dilute and carry away the gaseous impurities.

In laying the sewer or drain from the cesspool to the house, the precautions which Mr. Waring suggests should be taken to secure tight joints and a solid bed; a good running trap should be inserted not far from the house and iron soil-pipe from within the house carefully connected. Within the house, the soil-pipe itself should be independently ventilated by carrying its upper end out through the roof, and making an opening in its lower end in basement to complete the circulation. One or the other of these openings must be connected with the kitchen flue (in which there is always a fire), and the other with the outer air. Thus equipped, we have a system which is at least safe against the entrance of " sewer gas " by the ordinary channels. The existence of any pressure within the soil-pipes and drains is guarded against, and the system of ventilation provides for the constant dilution and removal of gaseous products of decomposition whether produced in the cesspool or soil-pipes.

The remaining sources of danger are from impure "ground air," and the vitiation of the local water. The latter is admitted as a fact, and the plan under discussion is recommended only where the water-supply is brought from a distant and untainted source. The former only need therefore be considered. Now, assuming a moderately pervious soil at the level of the bottom of the cesspool (and without this the cesspool soon becomes practically a tight one,) the purely fluid part of the sewage will probably travel a long way, indeed—*will mingle with the subterranean streams which exist in almost all localities.*

But it should be remembered that all of this sewage is usually enormously diluted with water, that we have provided for the removal of its more volatile constituents, and finally that the liquid portion in flowing away passes through what we may regard as a huge filter which washes out and retains the remaining organic constituents. So long as the surrounding soil is able to decompose and absorb the matter thus committed to it, no danger accrues. In the course of time, however, the capacity of the surrounding soil is exhausted; and the gases resulting from the decomposition of organic impurities begin to rise, unpurified and noxious, through the upper strata of the soil.

At first the absorbent and disinfectant powers of the latter will disarm the enemy; but ultimately the impure air and gases we have so much cause to dread will reach the surface, and mingle with the outer air. But when this is the case, are we any worse off than under the "subsoil" irrigation system? With that *all* the decomposition occurs at the surface of the ground, and dependence is placed on vegetation and free admixture of the air to neutralize its effects. But why are not the same means to be equally relied upon for neutralizing and dispersing the products of decomposition which may occur at a greater depth below the surface? Probably these products are diffused over a much greater area of ground on reaching the surface than they would be under the other system, and are already diluted and partially disarmed for harm.

One caution should be observed, however, where this plan is followed, particularly where the cesspool is not well removed from the house; namely, to guard against any possible rising of emanations from the ground *within the house*, by having well-cemented cellar walls and floor (or, better still, in addition to these, an open area around the house); but this precaution is one that ought to be observed with any system, and in all houses.

In conclusion let me say that the above plan is only suggested for houses "which stand on level ground," and which have a safe and abundant water-supply. For more favorably situated cases, better plans, no doubt, are available; but for the case I have supposed, I have seen none suggested by which at moderate cost equal safety can be secured. But in this correspondence I have been a seeker after knowledge, not an expounder of it; and I shall be glad to learn of better plans than that I suggested, if such there are.

T.

---

*January* 27, 1877.

MR. TOWNE instances the case of a house standing on level ground, such as prevails in the villages of Central New Jersey, and suggests the course to be pursued where the character of the surface makes it impossible to secure the requisite fall for the use of sub-irrigation drains. He supposes the case of " an ordinary house-lot, say fifty by a hundred and fifty." Let us suppose, by way of illustration, that the rear fifty feet of such a lot is to be used for the disposal of sewage by underground land-drain pipes. One of the conditions of the success of the system is that the slope shall not be too great. In arranging the sewerage of Lenox, Mass., where a large volume will be distributed, I have taken a fall of one in three hundred, or four inches to one hundred feet. For a private place where the wastes of a single household are to be accommodated, and where the flush-tank would not discharge more than from thirty to fifty gallons at a time, it would be better to have a fall of one in two hundred, or six inches to one hundred feet. More than this would be too much; and were the slope greater, I should propose to lay the lines on a course diagonal to the inclination of the land. The reason for this is, that if the inclination is greater, the flow runs too rapidly to the far ends of the lines, instead of leaking out more equally at each joint of its course.

To provide a fall of one in two hundred on the rear fifty feet of a level lot, would require a slope of only *three inches*, which could be made by handling an average depth of one and a half inches over the whole, or only about three hundred cubic feet of earth—an amount less than the ordinary modifications in grade of any tolerably finished house-lot. Indeed, a part of the slope required could be given in the drains themselves, as there probably would be no disadvantage in making them a little more or a little less than twelve inches deep at their ends.

I trust that this explains my statement that there is no practical difficulty in arranging for the application of this system, even on level ground. Of course, provision must be made to deliver the soil-pipe, or the outlet of the flush-tank, at a point sufficiently high to reach these drains; but there is not the least difficulty in doing this. The question of cost, so far from being "ignored," is a leading argument in favor of the irrigation-drain system; for in no other way, even on level ground, can the problem be so cheaply solved.

Mr. Towne's suggestion for a leaching cesspool is simply inadmissible. I am confident that no sanitarian, who has kept himself at all well informed of the progress of knowledge on this subject would permit the use of this device. The suggestions for the construction and ventilation of such a cesspool are practical and good in their way; but the objection to it is radical, and cannot be overcome. There are many conditions where, so far as the immediate occupant of the house is concerned, no harm may be done; and of course in the country, where the excavation is made at a distance from any probable future house site, there is less to be said against it. But in any congregation of houses in a town or village, the public authorities should strictly prohibit any such fouling of the earth.

If the soil is so tight that there is no leaching, then, however loose the wall, there is no escape of the liquid. If through sand, gravel, porous strata, fissures in rock, or any other means of escape, the liquid soaks away, we may be quite sure that it will carry filth to greater and greater distances as time goes on ; and, as the soil becomes foul, it will retain the objectionable or dangerous ingredients. Deep down in the earth, away from the action of the atmosphere, we lose the effect of the cleansing oxidation of the air, and of the action of roots, which are the best agents in purifying all manner of sewage. In fact, the objection is a radical one.

We cannot safely retain on our premises a putrefying mass of organic filth; and our own safety, and the safety of the community, require that we shall not pour this filth into unknown subterranean recesses, from which it may taint the water of the wells and the ground-air under houses.

Mr. Towne suggests the cementing of cellar floors as a safeguard against the rising of foul air into the house. To accomplish this end, such cementing must be absolutely tight, and the same tightness must be given to the surrounding wall. Both of these conditions are important to the best building, but they are often neglected for the sake of economy. So far as the drainage question is concerned, they would cost much more than would the adoption of the irrigation-drain system, even including the slight modification of grade that this might make necessary.

Mr. Towne asks, Why are we worse off with the exhalations from leaching into the deep soil (and under our houses) than with the irrigation system where the whole of the decomposition takes place close on the surface of the ground?

Precisely because of the difference between a decomposition taking place in the absence of fresh air and roots and the rapid and destructive process which these agencies insure. The most serious evils may result from the putrefaction of organic matters stored in large masses, or closely covered from the air. The same materials consumed by the concentrated oxygen of aerated earth, especially when an active vegetation stands ready to take up the results of the decomposition, produce no hurtful result.

W.

*February* 3, 1877.

THE communications printed in a recent issue of your journal, from Mr. Waring, jun., and Mr. Towne, discussing the drainage of houses on level ground, have raised a question of great interest, and I ask permission to say a few words on the same subject.

There are situations and conditions which render practicable the system of house-drainage preferred by Col. Waring, which disposes of the liquid waste of the house by means of flush-tanks, settling cisterns, and irrigation-pipes. I have employed this system, somewhat modified, in draining my own country house, which stands on high ground, and has a sloping lawn of more than a hundred feet width, in the best position for the accommodation of irrigation pipes. I do not believe, however, that the system is one which admits of general adoption, nor one which will meet the requirements of most householders living within the narrow limits of town or village lots. Even where practicable, it does not seem to me to possess the theoretical excellence which is claimed for it. In summer, when evaporation is rapid and vegetation active, it is possible that the organic matter in the waste of a house would be taken up and assimilated by plants as rapidly as it could decompose in the soil; but I am not quite sure that even this is true in all soils.

I have watched very carefully the workngs of the system in my own grounds; and while the lines of drain-pipe are laid within eighteen inches of the surface, which is quite even, I have failed to discover any indications of a more rapid or luxuriant growth of grass or weeds near the pipes than remote from them. If, however, it be conceded that the system works well in summer under average conditions, I fail to see that my buried pipes are much—if any—better than a leaching cesspool during the winter months, when the ground is frozen and vegetation dormant.

During this time the ground surrounding, and particularly that underlying the pipes, becomes charged with impurities which it cannot dispose of in a legitimate way. Long before they can be appropriated by growing plants, thawing snows and soaking rains carry these impurities deep into the soil where the plants cannot reach them. In a light porous soil there is nothing to hinder these accumulations of six or seven months of each year from working down until the soil is saturated and our own or our neighbors' well polluted. We have, in the Northern States, only about five months of warm " growing-weather "; and in my judgment, draining into the soil during the other seven months means pollution of the soil.

From a careful study of the problem of house-drainage in unsewered neighborhoods, I am satisfied that the tight cesspool system is the only one which is practicable. I have many times during the past few years had occasion to recommend a plan of drainage which has the advantage of adaptation to all the conditions I have yet encountered in practice. It is neither an invention nor a discovery; but in these matters the attainment of good results is of much more consequence than novelty or ingenuity in the means employed. I contract with a responsible mason to build a cesspool as "tight as a bottle." The price depends somewhat upon circumstances; but as I select my mason and give him to understand that he is to estimate honestly on the cost of first-class materials und workmanship, and not as a competitor for a contract to be given to the lowest bidder, the price is usually reasonable and the work always good.

When there is plenty of room, I put the cesspool from fifty to sixty feet from the house; when the lot is small, I put it as far away as I can. In shape the cesspool is much like an old fashioned coffee-cup; its size, taking an average, is five feet diameter at top, and six feet deep. I cover this with a stout platform, removable at will, from the middle of which rises a wooden chimney ten or twelve inches square in cross section, and three to five feet high, capped with one of Mr. Baldwin Latham's charcoal ventilators, or with a device embodying the same principle. At one side of the platform I set a pump—any one of several makes is adapted to the purpose— and run the suction-pipe down to the bottom of the cesspool. This pump is a permanent fixture, and is always ready for use. The house connection is made in the usual way; but I have no traps at any point on the line of the main waste or soil-pipe, or the house-drain proper. The soil-pipe is carried up of one size from the foundation wall to and through the roof. The branch waste-pipes are of course trapped; but I take the precaution to use traps which cannot lose their seals from any cause except evaporation. The danger to be apprehended from the absorption and transmission of cesspool gases by the water-seal of such traps is obviously very slight, at most. With the house-drainage system open at both ends, no accumulation of gases at any point where they can be held under pressure is possible.

When the cesspool is full, it can be emptied in any way most convenient. In a town or village where an odorless excavator can be ordered, it may be emptied by lifting out the ventilating chimney, and dropping the suction-pipe of the apparatus through the hole in the platform. If the householder must attend to the work himself, he can do it in one or two ways, according to circumstances. In summer, if he has a garden, he may employ it for surface-irrigation. He can make a trough by nailing two boards together at right angles, and, putting one end of this under the spout of his pump, let the other end rest where the water will do most good. By providing two or three such troughs made of long boards, he can irrigate a garden of considerable extent, and as frequently as may be needed. The organic matter already partially decomposed will be at once taken up by the plants; and the water is quickly absorbed by the dry surface soil, to be given off again in evaporation. In the winter, or in places where irrigation is not needed for the fertilization of a well-kept garden, the contents of the cesspool must be pumped into tight vessels of some sort, and carried away. A short piece of rubber tubing attached to the spout of the pumps, and half a dozen kerosene-barrels with tight-fitting bungs, will give the householder an odorless excavator of his own.

Concerning the views expressed by my very intelligent friend Mr. Towne, I can only say that, in my judgment, the leaching cesspool system is the worst which can be employed under any circumstances. I lately visited a town in which this system is carried out *par excellence*. The town is built upon a limestone foundation, which is full of cracks and fissures.; and, to dispose of anything in the shape of waste, it is only necessary to dig down twenty or thirty feet, until the limestone is reached. Even privy-vaults empty themselves. The town has a water-supply drawn from sources not reached by the pollution of the soil; but within three years it has had two epidemics of typhoid fever, and is never free from sickness of unmistakable zymotic origin. We must not forget that, in pouring sewage into the soil, we are poisoning it for the future, near and remote. Coming generations will suffer, even if we do not, the consequences of so reckless a disregard of the precautions which the experience of centuries has shown to be essential to the avoidance of conditions prejudicial to the public health.

B.

NEW YORK, *Jan.* 22, 1877.

---

*March* 10, 1877.

I WAS much interested in the courteous responses of Col. Waring and Mr. Towne to my letter on the drainage of country houses, published in your issue of Feb. 3, and regret that I could not find time for an immediate reply.

I cannot wholly agree with Col. Waring's views respecting the absorptive and oxidizing power of the soil, without taking certain well defined exceptions to his very general conclusions. A full discussion of the points at issue must be more appropriate to the columns of an agricultural journal than to one devoted to architecture; but as architecture and drainage are of necessity closely allied, the subject possesses a practical interest for a very large proportion of your readers.

In my judgment, formed after some observation, the adaptation of the soakage system to house drainage depends upon a variety of conditions, primarily upon the character of the soil. If I attach more importance to the action of vegetation than Col. Waring does, he attaches more importance to the powers of the soil and its contained oxygen than I do. In his communication published in your issue of Jan. 27, he speak of the "concentrated oxygen of aerated earth." I have never found any satisfactory evidence of the fact that oxygen is concentrated in the soil. Oxidation is unquestionably promoted by looseness of the soil; but this same condition favors the escape of gases resulting from the decomposition of organic matter, and those most productive of disease are not, so far as I know, appropriated by vegetation. In assuming that the character of the soil is of secondary importance as concerns the efficiency of the soakage system, Col. Waring seems to contradict himself. Very little air permeates a stiff clay soil, as he practically admits. Heavy clay soils do not in themselves exert a stronger absorptive action than porous soils. The absorptive powers of clay are only manifest when it is finely divided, as when burned or intimately commingled with the looser components of a light loam.

The experiment of straining dung-liquor through soil does not prove much, if anything, as regards the subject under consideration. The solid matter is simply removed by the ordinary process of filtration, and under the combined influence of heat, moisture, and air, it would quickly ferment. That "Organic matter once seized upon by the soil is never again given up in an unchanged condition," is not, I think, established. I know of one case where carrots planted in ground fertilized with material freshly removed

from an old privy-vault, were wholly unfit
for food. Washed clean and cut with a
knife, they were unhealthy in appearance
and offensive in smell. As to the "un-
yielding grip of the interior surfaces of
the soil to prevent added organic matter
from working downward," I fear there is
some room for doubt. It is certainly difficult to reconcile the proposition with the
fact that the roots of plants follow the
deposition of organic matter, and as in the
deepened soil of the Mapes' farm in New
Jersey, extend to twice the depth usually
reached by the roots of such plants. in
stiff soils, manifestly because the manure
had worked down as the depth of the soil
was increased.

There is a limit to the absorptive powers
of every thing. Even charcoal has its
limits, although its powers are to some
extent self-renewing. So it is with the
soil. When the surface is ice-bound there
is little opportunity for aeration. If un-
frozen below, it is likely to be sodden
from preceding rains, and under such cir-

cumstances the destruction of organic matter by oxidation would proceed but slowly.

That sewage can be discharged into the soil continuously, without ultimately polluting it to considerable depth and beyond the reach of the oxidizing influence of the air, I cannot believe. It is no uncommon thing to find deep wells polluted by impurities carried down from the surface. The water of wells sunk near barnyards is often unfit for use, even when danger of contamination by the flow in of unfiltered surface-water is effectually guarded against. On this point the experiments of Dr. Lissauer, as translated from *Deutsche Vierteljahr schrit* in the Proceedings of the Institution of Civil Engineers, are not without interest. The results of fifty-one experiments to determine the absorptive power of soils point to the following conclusions, among others:—

"1. The liquid entering the pores of the soil displaces the air or liquid previously present, forcing the former upwards into the atmosphere, and the latter downwards into the subsoil or effluent water.

"2. In order that the effluent water may not be directly polluted by the sewage liquid, the maximum supply of the latter must not be more than can be taken up by the pores of the soil.

"3. Dry, loamy soil absorbs more than peaty soil and gives up less, whilst dry sandy soil, on the contrary, absorbs less and gives up more. Consequently a loamy soil, though it absorbs a large quantity of liquid, can seldom be irrigated; whereas a sandy soil, though it absorbs but little, may often be irrigated,

"4. The looser the soil, the easier watercourses are formed in it, and therefore the less can its maximum power of absorption be approached: otherwise the sewage liquid might penetrate the subsoil before the whole of the ground had been saturated.

"5. In order therefore that the effluent water may be protected from pollution, it is especially necessary that the absorptive power of the soil should be known; but the determination is of no value unless it be made in a sample in which the natural position of the particles of earth has been undisturbed."

I have no desire to place myself in a position of antagonism to the system favored and defended by Col. Waring in his several communications. I consider it good, but like all good things it probably has its limitations. It rests with the engineer and the architect to intelligently determine what these are.

In Mr. Towne's letter, I find some statements which indicate that he has reasoned from imperfect data. The consumption of water in cities is certainly no standard by which to judge the consumption per head in country houses depending upon wells and cisterns; and I refer him to Col. Waring's last letter for an estimate, which, though very liberal, is more nearly correct. As regards cesspool capacity, it must, of course, depend somewhat upon circumstances. A nine-hundred-gallon capacity is by no means an arbitrary standard. Speaking generally, it is safe to say that the smaller the cesspool the better, inasmuch as it requires to be emptied the oftener. The conservation of filth under conditions favorable to the exercise of its power for mischief is never desirable. Eternal vigilance is the price of good health; and I have yet to see a drainage system applicable to isolated country houses which can be left to take care of itself without sooner or later becoming a nuisance and a danger. I should never drain roofs or carry storm-water from any shedding surface into a cesspool which also received the house-waste; and the danger of overflow from this cause need not be taken into account.

B.

---

*March* 24, 1877.

MR. BAYLES intimates that the reasoning contained in my last communication was predicated on "imperfect data," for the reason that " the consumption of water in cities is certainly no standard by which to judge the consumption per head in coun-

try houses depending upon wells and cisterns"; and he refers to Col. Waring's
estimate as more nearly correct. My
statement gave an average consumption
per head per day of thirty-eight gallons;
while Col. Waring's (in referring to a case
in which "there is no public water-supply") was thirty gallons. But by reference
to my letter of Dec. 16, 1876, with which
this discussion commenced, Mr. Bayles
will learn that the question therein pro-
posed was that of "the disposition of sewage from a country house, where there is
no town drainage available, where the
surrounding grounds are level, and *where
there is a street water-supply.*" On these
data I maintain that my reasoning was
correct; and, indeed, my own observation
is to the effect that where there is an abundant water service, the average consumption per head is usually much more than
thirty-eight gallons daily.

The problem I originally suggested is
one of great importance; but I think it
has been somewhat lost sight of in some
of the recent communications. In my

own limited experience I know of four towns, the populations of which range from 3,000 to 10,000, in which a public water-supply has been introduced for years without any corresponding provision for the removal of sewage. Indeed even the city of New Haven, which has long had a water-supply, was only efficiently sewered within the past eight years.

Without discussion I will concede that these conditions are intolerable, that a sewerage system should be contemporaneous with a water service, and that the introduction of the latter should in many instances be legally prohibited unless accompanied by the former; but this does not alter the fact that in hundreds of places, precisely these most objectionable conditions obtain, and probably will obtain for years to come. The question I have asked is, How, under these conditions, *and at moderate cost*, can the average householder make himself most secure against zymotic diseases originating from decomposing sewage?

Mr. Bayles adds other pertinent objections to those I have previously made against the irrigation-system urged by Col. Waring as so universally applicable; and I think it must be conceded that this system cannot be extensively relied upon *for use on private grounds* of small extent, particularly in our Northern States. At the risk of appearing too confident in my own judgment, as opposed to that of persons who have made a much more thorough study of this subject than I have been able to, I will say further, that the alternative system to which Mr. Bayles has committed himself—viz., the use of tight cesspools—seems to be equally inadmissible, for the reasons stated in my letter published in your number of 17th ult.

This is eminently a case in which it is easier to make objections than to give advice; but the subject is one, the importance of which, although but little recognized, cannot be over-estimated; and I sincerely trust that its discussion in your columns may lead to a better solution of it than has yet been offered.

T.

*April* 14, 1877.

I TRUST that your readers are not tiring of this discussion, for—unlike Mr. Bayles —I think it quite as appropriate, even in its agricultural details, to an architect's as to a farmer's paper. The question as to the action of the soil, and of the air which it contains, upon organic impurities added to it, is equally important whether we are considering the effect of this action in preparing food for plants, or in removing conditions dangerous to health. It has its sanitary side, and so claims the attention of the architect—the practical sanitarian. It is to be understood that what I propose is not a "soakage" system, but something that stops so far short of saturation that in an extreme case, as per my communication, only about one volume of liquid is added, per day, to over three hundred volumes of earth. The importance attaching to the soil as an agent of disinfection is due to its known powers of absorption and to the oxidizing effect of its contained air. "Satisfactory evidence of the fact that oxygen is concentrated in the soil" is to be found in the recorded testimony of many investigators in the field of agricultural physics.

Prof. Johnson, of New Haven, says:* "The soil, being eminently porous, condenses oxygen. Blumtritt and Reichardt indeed, found no considerable amount of condensed oxygen in most of the soils, and substances they examined; but the experiments of Stenhouse and the well-known deodorizing effects of the soil upon fæcal matters leave no doubt as to the fact. The condensed oxygen must usually expend itself in chemical action. Its proportion would appear not to be large; but being replaced as rapidly as it enters into combination, the total quantity absorbed may be considerable. Organic matters and lower oxides are thereby oxidized. Carbon is converted into carbonic acid, hydrogen into water, protoxide of iron into peroxide. The upper portions of the soil are constantly suffering change by the action of free oxygen, *so long as any oxidizable matters exist in them*."

* How Crops Feed, p. 218.

Schubler says :* "The earths possess the remarkable property of absorbing oxygen gas from the atmospheric air, a phenomenon pointed out many years ago, by A. von Humboldt. . . . This property of the earths is confirmed almost without an exception, provided they be employed for this purpose in a moist state." In the experiments which he instituted, exposing one thousand grains of different earths for thirty days in vessels of fifteen inches cubic contents (15 inches of air containing 3.15 inches of oxygen) he found that sandy loam absorbed 1.39 inches of oxygen, clay loam absorbed 1.65 inches and garden mould absorbed 2.60 inches.

This looks very much like concentration. All authorities agree in ascribing this power of condensing oxygen (and other gases) to all materials very much in proportion to their porosity. As charcoal is very porous, this is usually taken as an illustration. Voelcker says : † "It [charcoal] possesses the power not only of

absorbing certain smelling gases, sulphur-
etted hydrogen and ammonia, but also of
destroying the gases thus absorbed; for
otherwise its purifying action would soon
be greatly impaired. It is very porous,
and its pores are filled with *condensed*
oxygen to the extent of eight times its
bulk.

"We have therefore, in charcoal oxygen
gas (which supports combustion or lights
fires) in a condensed or more active condition than in the common air which we
breathe. Hence it is that organic matter
in contact with charcoal is so rapidly
destroyed. The beauty of charcoal is that
the destruction takes place imperceptibly,
and that its power of burning organic
matter is continually renewed by the surrounding atmosphere so that it is a constant carrier of atmospheric oxygen in a
condensed state in its pores. The oxygen
that acts on organic matter and burns it
up is speedily replaced, and the process
goes on continually. Hence it is that a
comparatively small quantity of wood or

peat charcoal is capable of destroying a very large quantity of organic matter."

Johnson, after describing and illustrating this action of porous substances, says:* "The soil absorbs putrid and other disagreeable effluvia, and undoubtedly oxidizes them like charcoal, though perhaps with less energy than the last-named substance, as would be anticipated from its inferior porosity." Jamieson says,† "All porous bodies which offer a considerable surface to gases act like charcoal." Saussure says that charcoal absorbs nine and a quarter times its bulk of oxygen. Prof. Way says:‡ "The reason that the sand accelerates the fermentation of the urine is no doubt this: all bodies possess a surface attraction for gases, and of course therefore for common air. This attraction, *which enables them to condense a certain quantity of air on their surfaces*, is in direct relation to those surfaces." Way

* How Crops Feed, pp. 170, 171.
† Journal Royal Agricultural Society, vol. xvii., p. 448.
‡ Journal Royal Agricultural Society, vol. xi., p. 366 *infra*.

filtered sewer-water through six inches of soil. In two and a half hours he collected half a gallon, which he analyzed. It contained no potash, "no ammonia or nitrogen in any form." The original liquid contained over three hundred grains to the gallon of organic matter and salts of ammonia." He found the *absorption* to extend to a weight of sewage-water *more than equal to the weight of the soil.* This, be it remembered, was an instantaneous mixture, with no opportunity for a constantly renewed oxidizing action.

That the soil absorbs the products of the decomposition of organic matter, and carries the decomposition to completeness, no chemist would question. This action is the basis of the efficiency of the earth-closet. In my own experiment, an analysis of the earth and ashes used in earth-closets for six years (probably ten times over) showed that practically all of the eight hundred pounds of solid dry matter estimated to have been deposited during the six years was destroyed by oxidation as completely as it would have been by actual burning in a furnace.

The investigations of Way and Thompson fully determine the *retention* of impurities by the soil—an action which they ascribe largely to the double silicates.

The porous condition of the soil does *not* favor the escape of gases. On the contrary, in the case of the earth-closet, dry and porous earth completely arrests the escape of gases, as is demonstrated both by the absence of smell, and by the absence of chemical reaction. If the quantity of decomposing matter is large and concentrated, gas may be formed in such volume as to force its way through, but *exhalation* does not occur. It is not claimed that the gases which are most productive of disease are appropriated by vegetation, but that they are destroyed by chemical action—by oxidation.

The report of Dr. Mouat, on the effect of the use of the earth-closet in the government institutions of India in time of cholera, is conclusive, at least so far as

this disease is concerned.* All recorded
evidence as to the use of the earth-closet
in stopping the spread of disease is to the
same effect.

I believe that I only "seem" to contradict myself. Loose soils are more freely
permeated by atmospheric air and heavy
clays are more retentive of organic impurities presented in solution. The air in the
loose soil oxidizes, and the double silicates
in the clay have other chemical action.
There is air in all soils sufficient to care
for the small amount of impurities discharged by a single household throughout
the mass, underlying twenty-five hundred
feet of surface; and there is clay enough
to have an important effect even in what
is called sandy loam.

The absorptive powers of clay are manifest to chemical tests even when solid
lumps of it are penetrated by solutions of
nitrogenous matter. I think my statement, that "organic matter once seized
upon by the soil is never again given up

*Twelfth Report of the Medical officer of the Privy
Council, pp. 104, 105.

in an unchanged condition," is the statement of an established fact—with the limitation that after the soil is *saturated*, it cannot "seize upon" new supplies until the first supply has become chemically changed. On the Mapes' Farm in New Jersey—where, by the way, I was a pupil in 1853—the manure was *ploughed* down, and the deposition of organic matter in the subsoil was mainly due to the decomposition of the roots of crops, which (like clover) have the power of deep penetration. In the clay subsoil of the richest and oldest garden, we find no evidence that organic matter has ever "worked down" into it; on the contrary, we know that, as "organic" matter, it does not do so even in nearly pure sand or gravel.

Of course "there is a limit to the absorptive powers of everything"—a limit to every thing, in fact,—but that limit in the soil is, in my opinion, very far beyond the needs of the case in hand. So, too, the "some extent" of the renewal of absorptive power is more than enough for the purpose. I believe that wells are polluted

by filth flowing through porous strata and
rock-fissures, not by filth that has once
been fairly *absorbed* by the soil.

The quotation from Lissauer applies to
*excessive flooding*, not to the limited discharge of sub-irrigation drains. Para-
graph (1) seems not opposed to my theory;
(2) applies obviously to much greater
flooding than is contemplated, as the effluent water at Merthyr Tydvil (less than one-
tenth as much land —loose and gravelly at
that—as I have recommended being used
per head) remains pure after the filter-bed
has been used for several years. (3) All
soils can be irrigated (with sewage?), but
heavy soils may not be so profitably irrigated because they part with their water so
largely by evaporation, and thus lose heat.
(4) We do not propose to tax the one-hun-
dredth part of the "maximum power of
absorption." (5) The limitation of our volume makes this inapplicable to the discussion. Of course the system of sub-irrigation has its limitations, but it is a vast step
ahead of any cesspool system.

If the experience of the world is of any

value, it is proven that the tight cesspool, which Mr. Bayles advocates, conserves filth under the conditons which are the *most* "favorable to the exercise of its power for mischief." Even eternal vigilance will not stop the putrefaction of its contents. With some experience and observation in such matters, I do not hesitate to express the opinion that the sub-irrigation system may be more nearly left to itself than any other I know about.

I can only answer Mr. Towne's question by repeating the opinion before given—that the sub-irrigation system is much the simplest, the safest, and the best; and that its cost is really trifling, even where the water from the kitchen sink, and the laundry trays in the cellar, has to be lifted with a pump to the level of the drains. He accepts, apparently, without question, the wrongly based objections of Mr. Bayles, and says, "I think it must be conceded that this system cannot be extensively relied on *for use on private grounds*, of small extent, particularly in our Northern States." To offset this, I can point to instances of success on such grounds in such localities, especially to my own, which has worked *perfectly*, Winter and Summer, for seven years. I have never heard of a case of failure. These examples, supported by the arguments give above, must sustain the claims of the sub-irrigation disposal of liquid house wastes, or those claims cannot be sustained by my advocacy.

Since writing the above I have found in an editorial of the *Agricultural Gazette* (London), of March 19, the following :

" The astonishing power of an aerated and porous soil and sub-soil (our knowledge of which we owe to Dr. Frankland) may be trusted a great deal more than engineers appear to trust it. Mr. Norman Bazalgette labored hard the other evening to prove that Merthyr filter-beds had done nothing like the work which Dr. Frankland had declared them capable of doing. But the answer to his criticism, which was given in the subsequent discussion, seemed to us complete; and as upon it rests the safety of the cheaper method which in the agricultural interest we recommend, we reproduce it here.

"At the close of his clear and conclusive argument on this subject, Dr. Frankland put the matter thus: 'I have analyzed the effluent water from the Merthyr filter-beds when only 230 people drained on to them per acre, and again when 500, and when 1,250 people were draining on to them per acre; and deducting and discounting the dilution by the subsoil water, in the first case it was thirty times as clean and as pure as it needed to be; in the second cases it was purified seventeen times more than enough; and in the last case, it was still three or four times purer than was necessary. Is it unreasonable, then, to believe that those filter-beds could have cleansed sufficiently or even more than enough the sewage of three or four times as many as the greatest of these numbers, if only the work had been given them to do.

"Now we contend that the work was given them to do, and that they did it." Then follows an explanation of the irregular distribution of the sewage over different parts of the ground, showing that although each area of about one acre received its due proportion of sewage, " the quarter of the plat which was next to the carrier had its full work to do from the first and till the last of its six hours' period; but it often was not till two or three hours had elapsed, that the quarter farthest from the feeder was even fairly wetted. And thus it was that while it may be true enough, that it was only the sewage of 20.000 people that was dealt with by the twenty acres of filter-bed at Troedyrhiew —being at the rate of 1000 people per acre —yet at least one-half, probably much more than one-half, of that beautifully purified effluent water must have come from areas of the filter-bed, which were being watered at the rate of 2,000, 3,000, or 4,000 people per acre."

My recommendation for the use of soil for the purification of household sewage was based on a calculation of only 175 people per acre. It is proper to explain that when Dr. Franklin says, that the

water was made " thirty times as clean
and pure as it needed to be," he means
thirty times purer than the Rivers' Pollution Commissioners' standard of fair po-
table water.

W.

www.ingramcontent.com/pod-product-compliance
Lightning Source LLC
Chambersburg PA
CBHW030614270326
41927CB00007B/1169